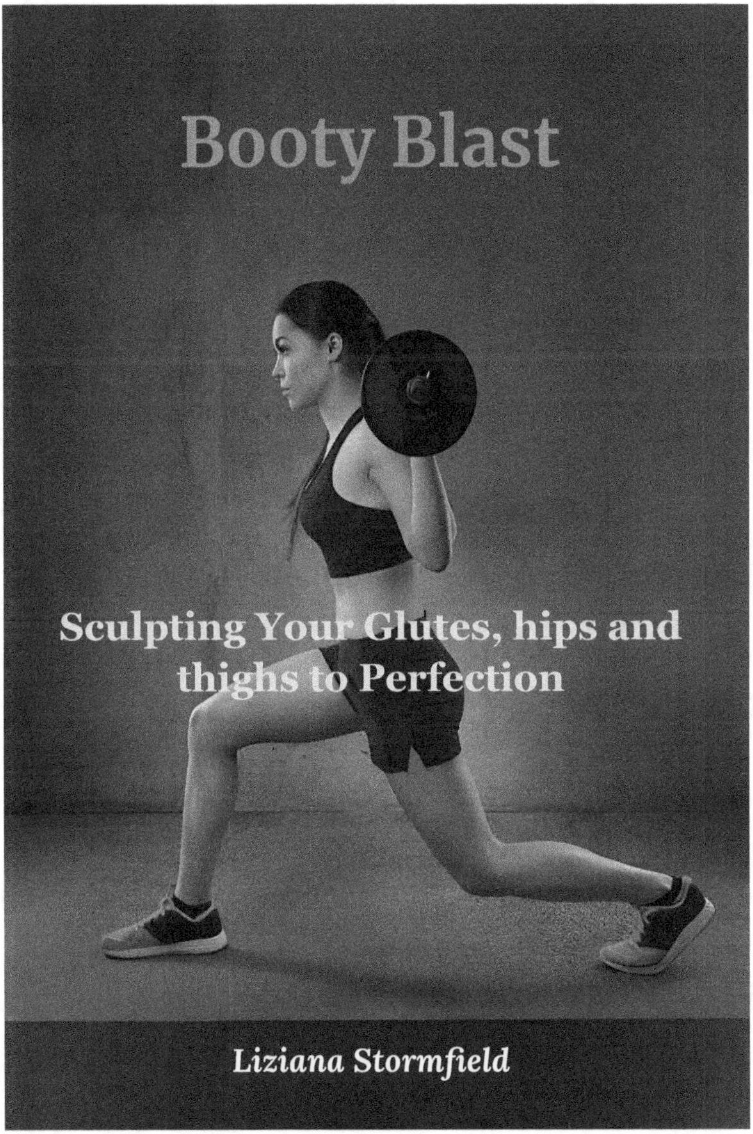

Booty Blast

Sculpting Your Glutes, hips and thighs to Perfection

Liziana Stormfield

Table of contents

Introduction

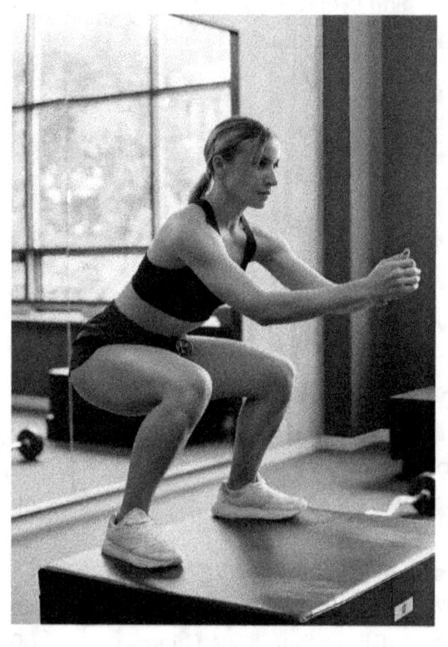

The glutes, hips, and thighs are the lower body's powerhouse, playing an important role in all of our daily motions and activities. These muscle groups are required not just for functional activities such as walking, jogging, and climbing stairs, but also for athletic performance and general body strength.

The gluteal muscles, which include the gluteus maximus, gluteus medius, and gluteus minimus, are the major muscles in the buttock area. They control hip extension, abduction, and rotation, which is critical for maintaining an upright posture and stabilizing the pelvis. The hip flexors, adductors, abductors, and rotators allow for a variety of hip joint movements such as flexion, extension, abduction, adduction, and rotation. These muscles support the pelvis and trunk, allowing us to walk, run, and squat.

The thighs are made up of the quadriceps, hamstrings, and adductor muscles. The quadriceps, positioned on the front of the thigh, are responsible for knee extension and are heavily used in activities such as walking, running, and jumping. The hamstrings, positioned on the back of the thigh, assist to bend the knee and extend the hip, which is essential for actions such as sprinting and bending forward. The adductor muscles on the inner thigh help to draw the legs together while also contributing to stability and balance.

Importance of Glute, Hip, and Thigh Workout

Imagine your body as a well-tuned machine, with each muscle group contributing significantly to its overall performance. Think of your glutes, hips, and thighs as the powerful engine that propels this machine forward. Just as a car needs a powerful engine to move forward, your body relies on these muscles to get you through life's obstacles and adventures.

Your glutes, hips, and thighs are more than just attractive; they are also strong, stable, and functional. They serve as the basis for your lower body, supporting you in activities such as walking, running, squatting, and jumping. Without a solid basis, even the simplest chores can become difficult and stressful.

However, usefulness is not the only consideration; performance is also important. Whether you're an athlete wanting to better your game or just want to move with comfort and elegance, focusing on these muscle groups can make a big difference. Strong glutes provide you the ability to sprint faster, jump higher, and lift more. Stable hips can boost your balance and agility, making you more nimble and responsive. Toned thighs not only look beautiful, but they also provide the strength and endurance required to take on any physical task.

Furthermore, a well-rounded training plan that includes glute, hip, and thigh movements will help you avoid injuries. Strengthening these muscles can help you avoid strains, sprains, and other common lower-body problems. This is especially important as we become older because maintaining muscular mass and strength is increasingly important for overall health and mobility.

So why wait? Begin including glute, hip, and thigh workouts into your program today to maximize the potential of your lower body. Whether you want to achieve peak performance or simply move with confidence and ease, these exercises will help you lay a solid, secure, and powerful foundation for a healthier, more active lifestyle.

Advantages of targeting certain muscle groups.

Targeting the glutes, hips, and thighs in a fitness plan provides numerous benefits that go beyond physical attractiveness. These muscular groups contribute significantly to overall lower body strength, stability, and mobility, affecting many facets of everyday life and athletic performance.

1. Improved Athletic Performance: Strong glutes, hips, and thighs are necessary for producing power, agility, and speed in sports and physical activities. Athletes in sports like running, jumping, and football rely

significantly on these muscles to perform explosive movements and quick direction changes.

2. Improved Functional Movement: The glutes, hips, and thighs are engaged in basic movements such as walking, jogging, and squatting. Strengthening these muscular groups enhances total functional movement, making daily tasks simpler and more efficient.

3. Injury Prevention: Weakness or imbalance in the glutes, hips, and thighs can result in a variety of injuries, especially in the lower back, hips, and knees. Targeted workouts serve to improve these weaknesses, lowering the likelihood of strains, sprains, and other ailments.

4. Improved Posture and Balance: Strong glutes, hips, and thighs help to stabilize the pelvis and spine. This can help with back pain and minimize the risk of falls, particularly in older persons.

5. Increased Metabolic Rate: Building muscle in these large muscle groups will help boost metabolism, assisting with weight management and fat loss. Muscles are

metabolically active tissues, therefore they burn more calories at rest than fat.

6. Improved Aesthetic Appearance: Targeted workouts can assist shape and tone the lower body, resulting in a more aesthetically pleasing figure. This can increase confidence and self-esteem.

7. Improved Bone Health: Resistance training, which is commonly used to target these muscle groups, can help boost bone density, lowering the risk of osteoporosis and fractures, especially in postmenopausal women.

Warm-up

The warm-up is an essential component of every fitness regimen, laying the groundwork for a safe and productive activity. Its major function is to prime the body for more severe action by raising heart rate, blood flow, and muscle temperature. A well-designed warm-up not only lowers the chance of injury but also improves performance and mental focus while exercising.

Benefits of Warming Up

1. Increased Muscle Temperature: Warming up gradually raises muscle temperature, making it more pliable and less susceptible to harm. This also improves muscular suppleness and contractility, which boosts performance and reduces the likelihood of strains or rips.

2. Improved Circulation: Performing mild aerobic activity during a warm-up increases blood flow to the muscles, providing the oxygen and nutrients needed for peak performance. This also aids in the elimination of

waste products generated during exercise, such as lactic acid, hence reducing muscle soreness.

3. Increased Joint Flexibility: Including dynamic stretching and mobility activities in your warm-up will help you improve joint flexibility and range of motion. This can improve workout technique and reduce the risk of joint injury.

4. Mental Preparation: A warm-up allows you to psychologically prepare for the upcoming workout, increasing focus and motivation. This mental preparation can improve overall performance and compliance with the training regimen.

Activation Exercises to Prep the Muscles

1. Cardiovascular Exercise: Light aerobic activity, such as running, jumping jacks, or cycling, increases heart rate and stimulates blood flow to muscles.

2. Dynamic Stretching: Dynamic stretches involve moving body components over a full range of motion,

which helps develop flexibility and mobility. Leg swings, arm circles, and torso twists are among examples.

Leg swings

Leg swings are a dynamic stretching technique that improves flexibility and mobility in the hip flexors, hamstrings, and quadriceps. Here's how to accomplish them:

Forward Leg Swings:
- Stand up straight and grab a stable surface, such as a wall or a chair, for support.
- Swing one leg forth and backward in a fluid movement.
- Maintain your torso upright and engage your core for stability.
- Swing 10-15 times with each leg.

Side Leg Swings:
- Stand sideways on a stable surface, one hand on it for support.

- Swing your outside leg across your torso, then out to the side in a smooth motion.
- Maintain an erect posture and activate your core.
- Swing 10-15 times with each leg.

Tips:
- Begin with small swings and gradually extend your range of motion as you feel more comfortable.
- Keep the swinging leg loose while using the supporting leg for stability.
- To avoid muscle fatigue, do not swing the leg too vigorously.

Leg swings are an excellent way to warm up the lower body before a workout, but they must be performed with control and in a comfortable range of motion to avoid injury.

Arm Circles

Arm circles are a simple yet effective workout that can help you improve shoulder mobility and flexibility.

Here's how to perform arm circles:

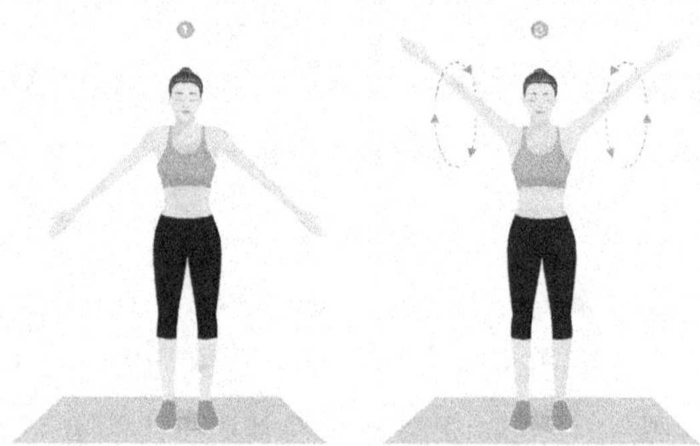

Stand tall with your feet shoulder-width apart and your arms straight out to the sides, shoulder height.

- Start by making small circular motions with your arms and progressively increase the size of the circles.
- Continue to rotate your arms forward for 15-30 seconds, then reverse direction and circle backward for another 15-30 seconds.
- Keep your shoulders relaxed and maintain a steady beat throughout the movement.
- Perform the exercise as needed to warm up your shoulder joints and increase flexibility.

Torso Twist

Exercises like torso twists are easy to do and very beneficial for increasing upper body mobility and flexibility. How to do them is as follows:

- Arrange your feet so that they are shoulder-width apart, and hold your arms straight out in front of you at shoulder height.
- Maintain an engaged core as you progressively rotate your torso to one side while maintaining your forward-facing hips.
- After a brief period of holding the twist, go back to the initial position.
- For a predetermined number of repetitions or amount of time, repeat the twist on the opposite side.

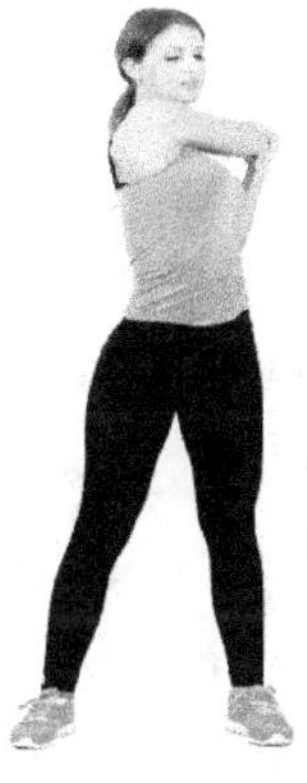

Torso twists are beneficial because they increase the range of motion and lower the chance of injury by assisting in the loosing of the muscles in your shoulders, core, and back. The muscles on the sides of your abdomen, known as the obliques, are also worked, which helps enhance stability and posture. To assist warm up your upper body for more strenuous activities and to increase general flexibility, incorporate torso twists into your warm-up regimen.

3. Activation Exercises: These exercises work on specific muscle groups to activate and prepare them for the next session. Glute bridges and bodyweight squats, for example, can activate the glutes and thighs before a lower-body workout.

4. Skill-Based Drills: Including skill-based drills in the warm-up for sports-specific workouts can help improve technique and prepare for the main activity.

Duration and Intensity:
A warm-up typically lasts 5 to 15 minutes, depending on the intensity of the workout and personal fitness level. The intensity should progressively increase, beginning with low-impact activities and progressing to higher-intensity motions.

Glute Exercises

Squat

Squats are an excellent workout for targeting the glutes, hips, and thighs. They can be performed in a variety of ways to accommodate different fitness levels and objectives. Here is a basic guide for performing squats and some frequent variations:

Basic squat:

- Stand with your feet shoulder-width apart, toes pointing slightly outward.
- Keep your chest elevated and your back straight.
- Lower yourself by bending your knees and pushing your hips back, as if you were sitting on a chair.
- Get as low as possible while keeping your heels level with the ground and your chest up.
- Push your heels back to the beginning position.

Variations:

1. Goblet Squat: When squatting, keep a dumbbell or kettlebell near your chest. This promotes equilibrium and increases resistance.

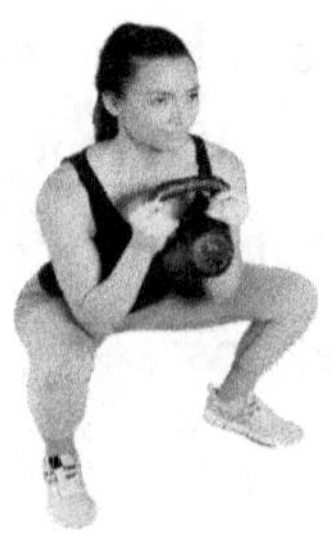

2. Sumo Squat:

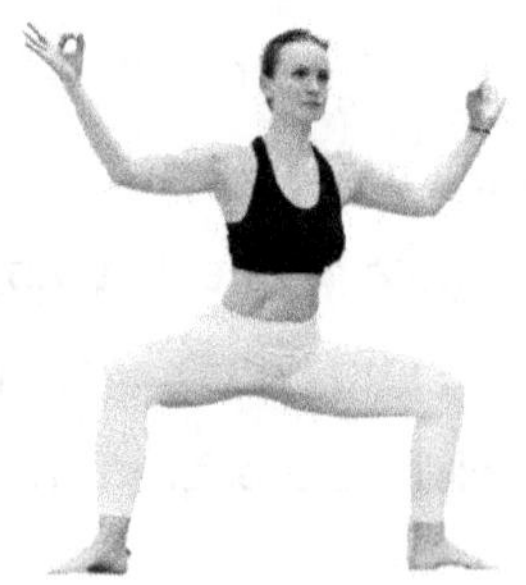

Stand with your feet wider than shoulder-width apart, toes pointing outward. Squat while paying special attention to your inner thighs.

3. Pulse Squat: Do a basic squat, but instead of returning to the starting position, pulse up and down slightly before rising.

4. Jump Squat: Squat down and then jump up explosively, landing softly back in the squat position.

5. Split Squat: Stand with one foot in front of the other and drop your body into a lunge before returning to the starting position.

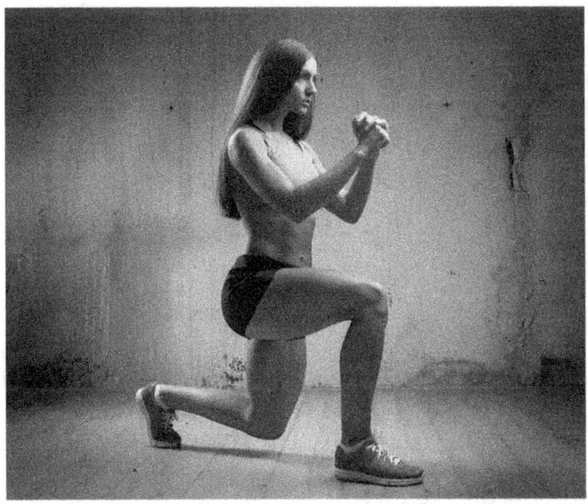

Technique Tips:

- Keep your core engaged throughout the action to protect your lower back.
- To avoid knee soreness, make sure your knees do not extend beyond your toes.
- Concentrate on pressing through your heels to activate your glutes and hamstrings.
- Maintain proper form by raising your chest and keeping your back straight.

Squats can help grow and tone your lower body, improve overall athleticism, and enhance functional movement. Begin with bodyweight squats and gradually increase weight, or try different variations to challenge yourself and keep your workouts interesting.

Lunges

Lunges are a terrific way to strengthen the legs and glutes. The steps are as follows:

Forward lunges:

- Stand with your feet hip-width apart.
- With your chest high and shoulders back, take a large stride forward on one leg.
- Make your front thigh parallel to the floor and bend your knees at a 90-degree angle.
- Lower your body to that stance.
- Reverse the method, first elevating one leg to the starting position, then the other.

Reverse lunges:

- Stand with your feet hip-width apart.
- Step back with one leg, lowering your torso until your knees are bent at approximately a 90-degree angle.
- Keep your front knee in line with your ankle, and your back knee slightly lifted off the ground.
- Reverse the method, first elevating one leg to the starting position, then the other.

Side lunges

- Stand with your feet hip-width apart, hands on your hips, or relaxed at your sides.
- Step to the right with your right foot while keeping your left foot in place.

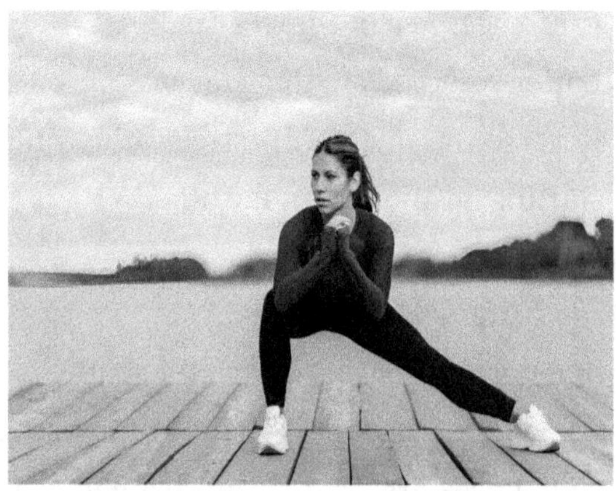

- Lower your body to the floor by bending your right knee and pressing your hips back, as if sitting in a chair.
- Keep your chest up and your left leg straight.
- To return to the starting position, push off with your right foot.
- Repeat on the opposite side, stepping with your left foot and lunging to the left.

- Repeat alternating sides for the appropriate number of times.

Keep your back straight, chest up, and core engaged throughout the exercise to preserve appropriate form and avoid injury.

Hip Thrust

Hip thrusts are a terrific exercise for the glutes, hips, and thighs. Here's how to execute them both with and without weights.

With Weight:

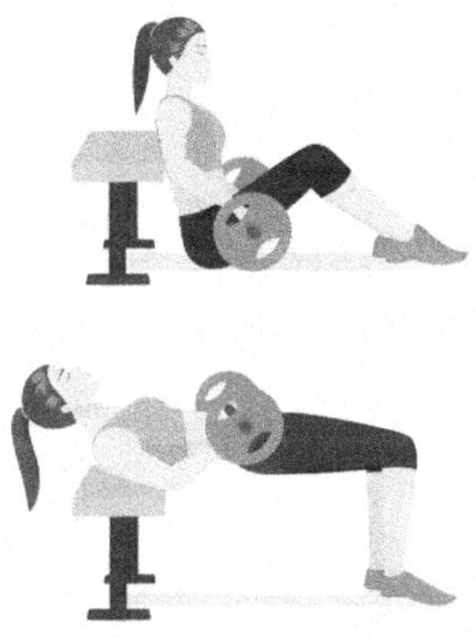

- Sit on the floor, with your upper back against a bench and a barbell over your hips.
- Roll the barbell over your legs and place it over your hips.
- Place your feet level on the floor, hip-width apart, and bend your knees at a 90° angle.
- Brace your core, grip your glutes, and push through your heels to raise your hips to the ceiling.
- When you reach the top, halt and gradually slide your hips back down.
- Repeat for the desired number of times.

Without Weights:
- Sit on the floor, with your upper back against a bench or higher surface.
- Bend your knees and place your feet flat on the ground, hip-width apart.
- To balance, place your hands on your hips or extend them out to the sides.
- Engage your core and glutes, then push through your heels to raise your hips to the ceiling.
- Squeeze your glutes at the top, then lower your hips down.

- Repeat for the desired number of times.

Tips:

- Maintain core engagement throughout the workout to protect your lower back.
- For best efficiency, squeezing your glutes at the top of the exercise is recommended.
- Begin with lesser weights or only your body weight, gradually increasing the load as you become more comfortable with the activity.

Glute Bridges: Basic and Advanced Techniques.

Basic Glute Bridge:

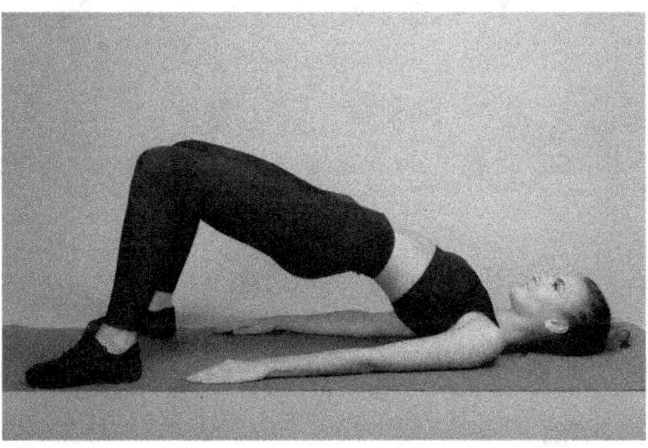

- Lie on your back, knees bent, and feet flat on the floor, hip-width apart.
- Tighten your core and glutes.
- Lift your hips off the floor so that your body forms a straight line from your shoulders to your knees.
- Hold for a few seconds before dropping your hips back to the starting position.
- Repeat the desired number of times.

Advanced Glute Bridge:

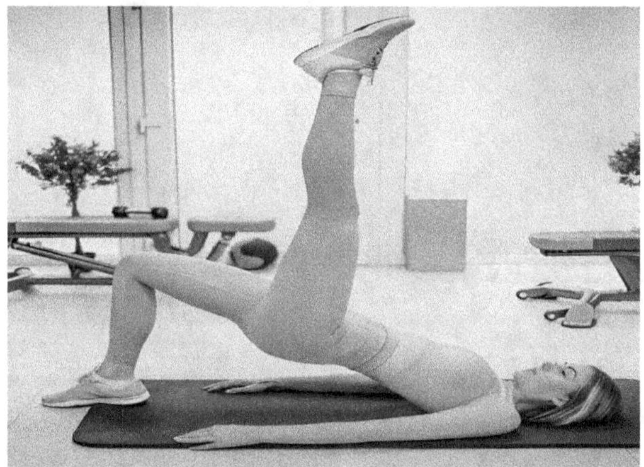

- Begin in the same posture as the Basic Glute Bridge.
- Lift one leg off the floor and extend it straight up to the ceiling.

- Engage your core and glutes, then lift your hips off the floor, only using the supporting leg.
- Hold for a few seconds before dropping your hips back to the starting position.
- Repeat with the opposite leg for the proper number of reps.

Tips for Both Variations:
- Engage your core throughout the workout to protect your lower back.
- To get the most out of the exercise, squeeze your glutes at the peak.
- To avoid arching your back excessively, keep your pelvis gently tucked under.
- Maintain control of the movement and avoid jerking or bouncing.

Benefits of Glute Bridges:
1. They strengthen the glutes, hamstrings, and lower back muscles.
2. Increase hip mobility and stabilization.
3. Improve athletic performance in activities such as jogging and leaping.

4. Help alleviate lower back pain by strengthening the muscles that support the spine.

Including glute bridges in your training routine will help you improve lower body strength, stability, and overall performance. Begin with the basic variation and gradually progress to the advanced form as you gain strength and confidence.

Deadlifts: Romanian and Sumo deadlifts

Deadlifts are an excellent exercise for strengthening your lower body and core. There are numerous types of deadlifts, including the Romanian deadlift and sumo deadlift.

Romanian Deadlift (RDL):
- Stand with your feet hip-width apart, holding a barbell or dumbbell in front of your thighs with an overhand grip.
- Keep your back straight, chest up, and shoulders back.

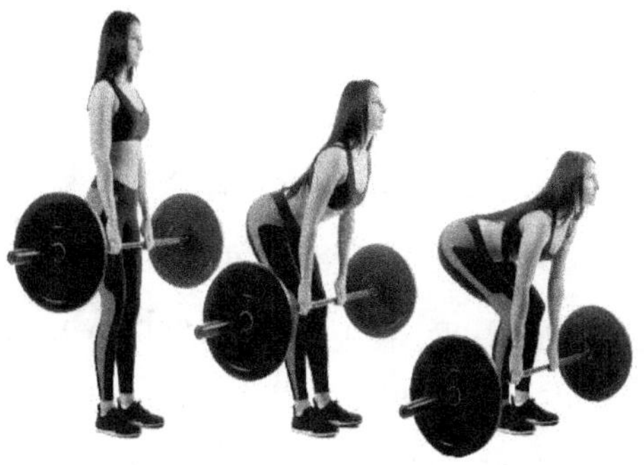

- Hinge at your hips and reduce the weight down the front of your legs while keeping it tight to your body.
- Lower the weight until your hamstrings feel stretched, then tighten your glutes and push your hips forward to return to the starting position.

Sumo deadlifts

- Stand with your feet wider than hip-width apart, toes slightly pointing out, and grasp the barbell with your hands inside your knees.
- Keep your back straight, chest up, and shoulders back.
- Push through your heels to elevate the weight, keeping it close to your torso.

- At the height of the exercise, lock out your hips and knees before lowering the weight slowly.

Both variations of the deadlift work your glutes, hamstrings, and lower back. The Romanian deadlift focuses on the hamstrings and lower back, whereas the sumo deadlift concentrates on the inner thighs and glutes. Incorporating both types throughout your workout plan can help you gain total lower-body strength and muscle development.

Hip workout: Hip abduction and side leg lifts.

Hip abduction is a simple but effective exercise that works the muscles on the outside of your hips known as the abductors. This exercise, which may be done lying down or standing up, serves to increase hip abductors, and improve hip stability, and overall lower body strength.

To do side leg raises:

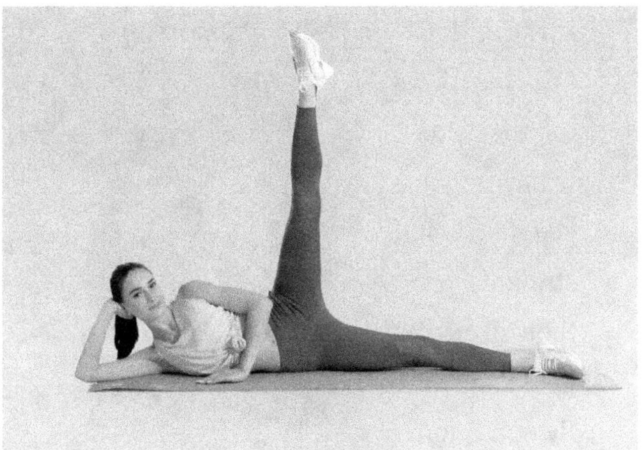

- Lying Down: Lie on your side, legs straight and piled on top of one another. Keeping your core engaged, bring your top leg up and away from your body as far as you can safely. Hold for a moment at the crest before lowering your leg back down. Repeat for the desired number of repetitions, then switch sides.

- Stand tall, feet hip-width apart. If necessary, maintain equilibrium by holding onto a sturdy surface. Lift one leg out to the side while keeping it straight, then drop it back down. Repeat on the opposite side.

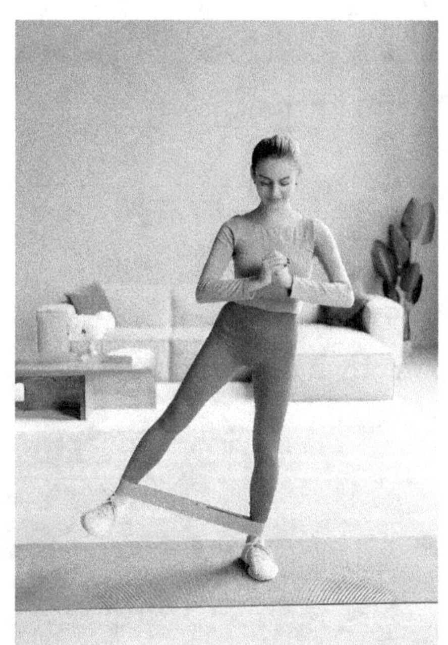

The Value of Side Leg Lifts

1. Strengthens Hip Abductors: The gluteus medius and minimus are two muscles that are particularly targeted by side leg lifts. In addition to minimizing the danger of injury and enhancing total lower body strength, exercising these muscles can aid improve hip stability.

2. Enhances Hip Mobility: You may enhance your hips' range of motion and flexibility by practicing hip abduction movements, which are required for actions like walking, running, and dancing.

3. Improves Balance and Stability: Having strong hip abductors helps people maintain higher balance and stability, which lessens their danger of falling, particularly when they're older.

4. Assists with Rehabilitation: Because hip abduction exercises strengthen the surrounding muscles and promote joint stability, they are usually prescribed as a

component of rehabilitation programs for injuries to the hip and knee.

By adding side leg lifts to your training plan, you can develop hip stability, mobility, and total lower body strength by targeting and strengthening the typically neglected hip abductor muscles.

Clamshells:

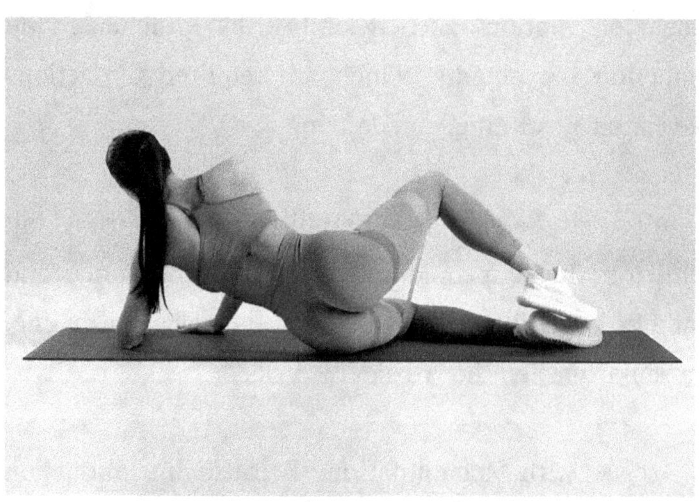

Another fantastic exercise for strengthening the gluteus medius and other hip abductors is the clamshell. How to execute clamshells:

- Lay on your side: To begin, put yourself on your side with your knees and hips bent 90 degrees. Place your feet in a stack on top of one another.

- Open your upper knee as much as possible without rotating your hips while maintaining your feet together. Your hip should contract as a result.

- Close your knee: Reposition your upper leg slowly to its initial position. After completing the required number of repetitions, move to the opposing side.

The significance of clamshells

Since the gluteus medius is typically weak in many persons, clamshells are significant. Enhancing the strength and function of the lower body can be achieved by strengthening this muscle, which can also minimize the risk of ailments like IT band syndrome and knee pain and promote hip stability.

Inner Thigh Leg Lift: A Workout for Toned Thighs

A simple but yet powerful exercise that works the adductor muscles of the inner thigh is the inner thigh leg lift. To complete this exercise, execute the following actions:

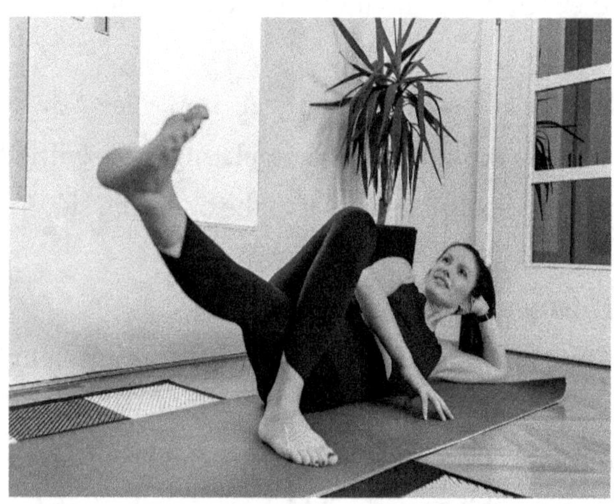

- Lie on your side: On a mat or other soft surface, begin by lying on your side. Make sure your complete body, from head to toe, is in a straight line.

- Set your legs up: Put your foot flat on the ground in front of your bottom leg, stretch your top leg, and bend your bottom leg. Your body will be more stabilized as a result of the training.

- Lift your lower leg: Lift your lower leg slowly toward the ceiling while maintaining a straight leg. Concentrate on elevating the leg with the muscles in your inner thighs.

- Lower your leg: Return your leg to the starting position gradually, maintaining your body in control the entire time.

- Repeat: As many times as you can without sacrificing good form, do ten to fifteen reps on each leg.

The Value of the Inner Thigh Leg Lift

1. Targeted Muscle Engagement: The inner thigh leg raise focuses on strengthening and training the adductor

muscles of the inner thigh, an area that is commonly disregarded.

2. Enhanced Leg Strength and Stability: You may enhance your entire leg strength and stability, which is useful for exercises like jogging, dancing, and walking, by strengthening your adductor muscles.

3. Improved Balance and Coordination: Exercises that focus on certain muscle groups, such as the inner thighs, can enhance general balance and coordination, minimizing the danger of accidents and falls.

4. Injury Prevention: Building stronger inner thigh muscles can assist avoid sprains and strains, particularly while engaging in activities that call for sudden direction changes or lateral movement.

5. Aesthetic Benefits: Sculpting and shaping the inner thighs can help give the body a more confident and gratifying image.

By integrating the inner thigh leg raise into your daily training regimen, you can lower your probability of injury, build stronger, more toned thighs, and boost overall leg strength and stability. To get the most out of the inner thigh leg raise and decrease the danger of strain or injury, technique counts just as much as with any other exercise.

Hip Flexors: Increasing Flexibility and Strength

Consider your hip flexors as the structure that connects your legs to your core and upper body. It's like having a rusty, creaky bridge that inhibits your range of motion when these muscles are weak or tight. However, you can turn your hip flexors into a strong, flexible bridge that supports you in every stride and movement by practicing the necessary stretches and strengthening exercises.

Stretching Your Hip Flexors: Unlocking the Door to Flexibility

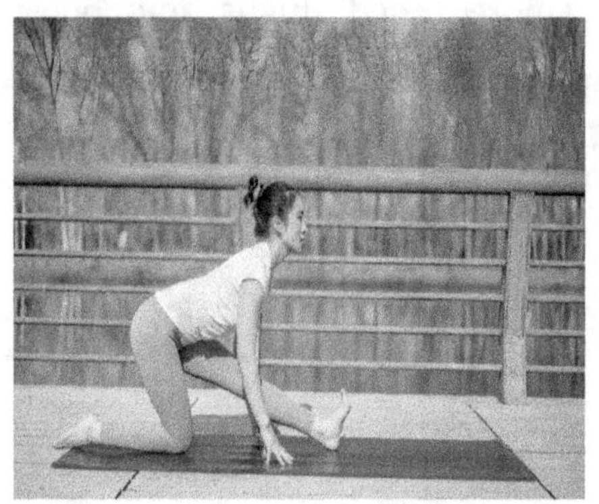

1.Place your other foot flat on the floor in front of you while you kneel on one knee. Maintaining a straight back, lean forward until you feel a stretch in the front of your hip. After 20 to 30 seconds of holding, switch sides.

2. Lying Hip Flexor Stretch: While lying on your back, extend one leg straight out and bend the other. Using a towel or band if required, carefully bring the outstretched leg toward your chest until you feel a stretch at the front of your hip. After 20 to 30 seconds of holding, switch legs.

3. Stunting the Hip Flexors: Take a tall posture, stepping one foot in front of the other. You should feel a stretch at the front of your hip after bending your back knee slightly and tilting your pelvis forward. After 20 to 30 seconds of holding, switch sides.

Strengthening Your Hip Flexors: Establishing a Strong Base

1. Leg Raises: Extend your legs straight out in front of you while lying on your back. Straightening one leg, raise it toward the ceiling and then slowly bring it back down. Do ten to fifteen repetitions on each leg.

2. Hip Flexor Bridge: Place your feet flat on the floor and your knees bent while lying on your back. Engage your core and squeeze your glutes as you raise your hips toward the ceiling. After holding for a short while, release the pressure. Repeat ten to fifteen times.

3. Lunges: Step one foot forward a long way, then drop your body until both knees are bent 90 degrees. Repeat on the other side after pushing yourself back up to the starting position. Try to do 10 to 15 repetitions per leg.

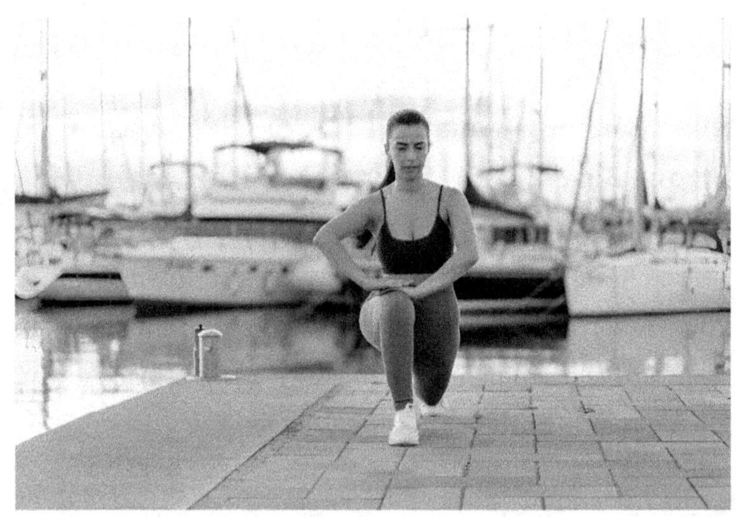

Hip Flexor Strengthening and Stretching Is Crucial:

1. Increased Flexibility: You can move more freely and effectively by stretching your hip flexors on a regular basis. This will increase your range of motion and flexibility.

2. Lower Risk of Injury: When engaging in activities that call for abrupt direction changes or explosive

movements, strong, flexible hip flexors can help lower the risk of injuries like strains or tears.

3. Enhanced Athletic Performance: You can improve your athletic performance in activities that call for running, jumping, or kicking by strengthening and extending your hip flexors.

4. Improved Posture: Bad posture can be caused by taut hip flexors. These muscles can be strengthened and stretched to help with posture, which lowers the risk of back discomfort and other related problems.

Stretches for the hip flexors and strengthening exercises will help you reach your body's maximum potential. These workouts can assist you in reaching your objectives and developing new levels of strength and flexibility, whether you're an athlete trying to enhance performance or just someone who wants to move more freely and pleasantly.

Thigh Workout

Leg Press: Different Foot Positions for Targeting Thigh Muscles.

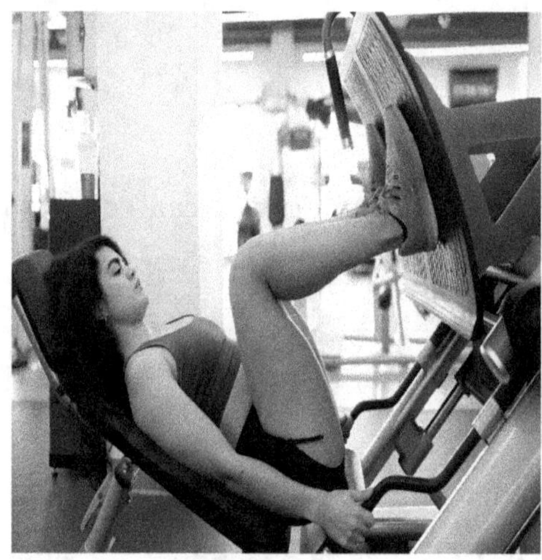

The leg push is a well-liked strength training exercise that works the hamstrings, glutes, and quadriceps, among other thigh muscles. You can more precisely target certain thigh muscle regions by changing the position of your feet on the footplate.

Position of the Feet:

Standard Position (Shoulder Width Apart): The quadriceps, hamstrings, and glutes are among the muscles of the thigh that are targeted when you place your feet shoulder-width apart. For newcomers, this is a good place to start.

2. Wide Stance: This stance emphasizes the activation of the inner thigh muscles (adductors) by placing your feet wider than shoulder-width apart. Additionally, this stance works the hamstrings and glutes more.

3. Narrow Stance: Bringing your feet closer together works the vastus medialis (the muscle that makes up the inner quadriceps) and the abductors, the outer thigh muscles. This position can enhance knee balance and stability.

4. High Foot Placement: Grasping the footplate higher works your hamstrings and glutes more so than your quads. Additionally, this position lessens the strain on the knees.

5. Low Foot Placement: The quadriceps muscles are highlighted when your feet are positioned lower on the footplate. Use caution when using this position as it

improves the range of motion and may put more strain on the knees.

Tips for proper form:

1. Throughout the exercise, keep your back flat against the backrest as a tip for proper form.

2. Verify that your knees do not extend past your toes and are in line with them.

3. Execute the exercise with control; do not lock out your knees at the peak.

4. Modify the weight based on your desired degree of fitness and strength.

Advantages of Various Foot Positions

- Muscle Targeting: You can target different thigh muscle groups by shifting your foot position, which promotes balanced muscular growth.

- Joint Health: By dividing the workload among several muscle groups and joints, using diverse foot postures can help lower the risk of overuse issues.

Strength and Power: Improving the strength and power of particular muscle groups can help to enhance overall lower body performance.

 With the leg press, you may target different parts of your thigh muscles by changing the location of your feet, making it a very versatile exercise. You can attain balanced muscle development and lower your chance of overuse issues by varying your leg press exercise. To get the most out of this exercise, always maintain perfect form and adjust the foot position according to your comfort level and goals.

Leg Extension: Appropriate Position and Muscle Activation

A common exercise that works the quadriceps muscles (found on the front of the thigh) is the leg extension. It's a fantastic method for toning and

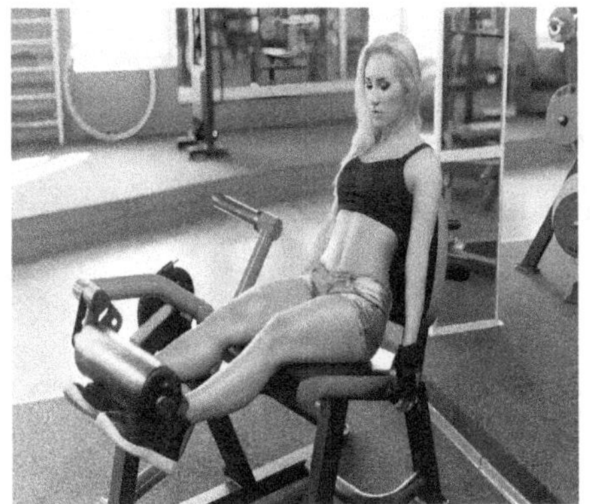

strengthening your legs, but to prevent injury and get the most out of your muscles, use the appropriate form.

Correct Form:

1. Set Up the Equipment: Take a seat on the leg extension machine with your feet hooked beneath the padded lever and your back flat against the backrest. Make sure your knees are parallel to the pivot point of the machine by adjusting the seat height.

2. Position Your Legs: Lay your thighs flat against the padded bar and rest your hands on the side grips for support. Your feet should be hanging off the side of the machine, and your knees should be parallel to its axis.

3. Execute the Movement: Extend your legs gradually until they are nearly straight, being careful not to lock your knees. Squeeze your quadriceps for a short while by holding the position, then gradually return the weight to the beginning position.

4. Controlled Movement: Throughout the workout, pay attention to moving slowly and deliberately. Steer clear of

momentum and swinging the weight, since these actions might decrease exercise effectiveness and raise the risk of injury.

5. Breathing: Exhale as you extend your legs and inhale as you decrease the weight. During the activity, this aids in maintaining appropriate breathing and core stability.

Muscle Engagement:

Quadriceps: The quadriceps is the primary muscle activated during leg extensions. The leg extension exercise primarily targets the muscle responsible for extending the knee, hence aiding in the strengthening and toning of the quadriceps.

Stabilizing Muscles: To support the movement and preserve good form throughout the leg extension exercise, other muscles, such as the calves and hamstrings, function as stabilizers. By using these muscles, you can increase the general strength and stability of your lower body.

Safety Advice: Use Appropriate Weight: As you get more accustomed to the activity, gradually increase from a small starting weight. Excessive weight usage might put a strain on your knees and raise the possibility of injury.

Prevent Locking Your Knees: Throughout the exercise, maintain a small bending in your knees to prevent locking them, which can put undue strain on your joints.

Pay Attention to Your Body: If you experience any pain or discomfort while exercising, stop right away and seek advice from a healthcare provider or fitness expert.

An effective exercise for toning and strengthening the quadriceps muscles is leg extension. You may optimize its benefits and lower your risk of injury by using the right technique and activating the right muscles. Include leg extensions in your exercise regimen to strengthen your lower body and raise your level of general fitness.

Squat Jumps: Use Plyometrics to Strengthen Your Thighs

Dynamic plyometric exercises like squat jumps can improve your lower body power and explosiveness while strengthening and toning your thighs. This exercise is a fantastic addition to any workout regimen that aims to improve athletic performance and build leg strength since it combines a basic squat with an explosive jump.

How to Do Jump Squats:

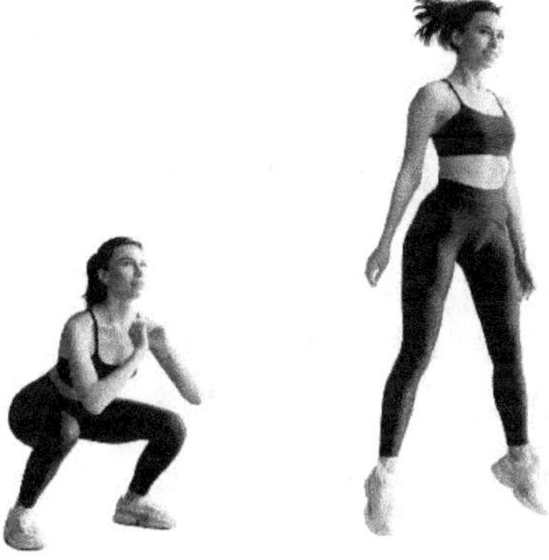

- Starting Position: Place your toes slightly outward while standing with your feet shoulder-width apart. Keep your core active and your chest raised.

- Squat: As you would if you were sitting back in a chair, bend your knees and push your hips back to lower your body into a squat position. Maintain your knees, crossing your toes, and your weight on your heels.

- Jump: Using your thighs and glutes, leap forward from a squat stance, fully extending your hips and knees. Elevate your arms to get momentum.

- Land: Bend your knees to cushion the impact as you gently land on the balls of your feet. To stay stable, keep your chest high and your core active.

- Repeat: Continue the squat jump for the predetermined number of repetitions or for the predetermined duration of time.

Advantages of Squat Jumping:

1. Thigh Muscle Strengthening: By focusing on the quadriceps, hamstrings, and glutes, squat jumps aid in toning and building these muscles.

2. Enhances Explosive Power: Squat jumps' explosive nature enhances your lower body power, which is advantageous for exercises like running and jumping that call for sudden bursts of energy.

3. Improves Athletic Performance: Squat jumps, whether you're a weekend warrior, basketball player, or runner, can improve your overall athletic performance by building lower body strength and power.

4. Burns calories: Squat jumps are an excellent complement to a weight reduction or fitness program since they are a high-intensity workout that can help burn calories and enhance cardiovascular fitness.

5. No Equipment Needed: Squat jumps are an easy exercise choice for at-home routines or on-the-go since they can be performed anywhere and don't require any equipment.

Safety Advice: As you get more accustomed to the exercise, start with fewer repetitions and progressively increase.

Pay attention to form to avoid injury. Retain your knees in line with your toes, and do not allow them to buckle inward.

To lessen the strain on your joints, land gently.

Squat jumps burn calories, strengthen and increase the power in your thighs, and enhance your athletic ability. They are a great addition to any fitness regimen. For a tough and efficient lower body workout, incorporate them into your leg day regimen or use them as part of a HIIT workout.

Wall Sits: Static Holding to Strengthen Thighs

Wall sits are a basic yet efficient way to build your thigh muscles, especially your quadriceps. This is a static hold workout, where you keep a particular position against a wall for a predetermined period.

How to Sit on the Wall:

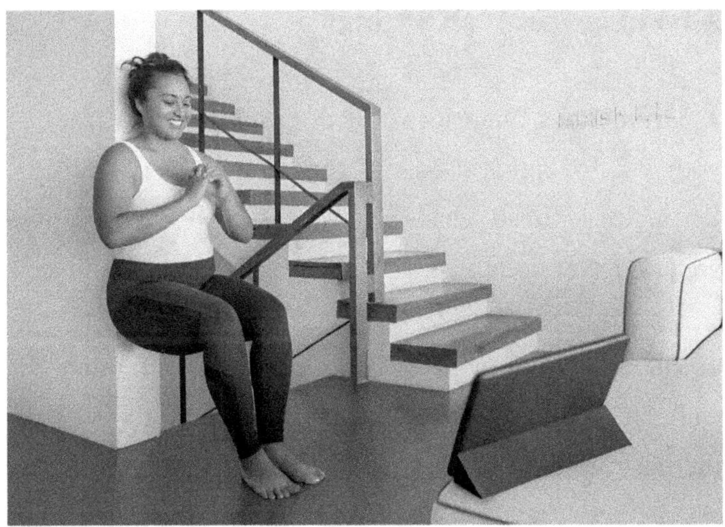

1. Locate a free wall space where you may rest your back against the wall without discomfort.

2. As if you were sitting in an invisible chair, slide down the wall until your knees are bent 90 degrees.

3. Keep your feet shoulder-width apart and flat on the ground.

4. Make sure your knees are exactly above your ankles, do not extend past your toes, and be sure that your back is flat against the wall.

5. Maintain this posture for as long as you can; for beginners, aim for 30 to 1 minute; as you gain strength, progressively extend the time.

Advantages of Wall Sitting:

1. Strengthens quadriceps: The muscles on the front of your legs, or quadriceps, are the main focus of wall sits. By making these muscles stronger, you can promote general lower body strength and enhance knee stability.

2. Increases Lower Body Endurance: Maintaining the wall sit position for a longer amount of time might increase muscle endurance, reducing fatigue during regular activities.

3. No Equipment Needed: Wall sits are an easy workout choice because they can be performed anywhere there is a clear wall area.

4. Low Impact: People with knee or hip problems can benefit from this workout because it is low impact, which means it places less strain on your joints.

5. Easy to Modify: By carrying weights or adjusting your leg position (e.g., one-legged wall sits), you can intensify wall sits.

Tips for doing wall sits:

1. To avoid knee discomfort, focus on proper form. Make sure your knees are aligned with your ankles and not bulging past your toes.
2. Keep your back flat against the wall during the exercise.
3. To remain calm and focused, breathe deeply and evenly while keeping the pose.

You can incorporate wall sits into your workout routine as a standalone exercise or as part of a lower body circuit. Begin with shorter intervals and gradually increase as you build strength and endurance. Include them 2-3 times each week for best results.

By incorporating wall sits into your routine, you may increase the strength and endurance of your thigh muscles, resulting in improved total lower body strength and function.

Cool Down

Stretching Routine

Stretching is an essential part of every workout routine, particularly when targeting the glutes, hips, and thighs. A daily stretching routine can assist improve flexibility, mobility, and range of motion in these major muscle groups, lowering the risk of injury and increasing overall performance.

Benefits of Stretching:

1. Improved Flexibility: Stretching allows muscles to extend and relax, increasing their flexibility. This can improve posture, minimize muscle stress, and boost athletic performance.

2. Increased Range of Motion: Consistent stretching can increase the range of motion in your joints, allowing for more fluid motions and reducing the risk of ailments like strains and sprains.

3. Reduced Muscular Soreness: Stretching after a workout can help reduce muscular soreness and stiffness by increasing blood flow to the muscles and assisting in the removal of lactic acid buildup.

4. Improved Posture: Tight muscles can lead to poor posture. Stretching can help to loosen these muscles, allowing you to maintain a more upright and natural posture.

Stretching Routine for the Glutes, Hips, and Thighs

1. Glute Stretch: Sit on the floor, one leg bent and the other stretched. Cross the ankle of the bent leg over the thigh of the stretched leg. Lean forward from the hips until your glutes feel stretched. Hold for 30 seconds then switch sides.

2. Hip Flexor Stretch: Kneel on one knee and place the other foot flat on the floor in front of you. Lean forward

with your back straight until you feel a stretch in the front of your hip. Hold for 30 seconds then switch sides.

3. Hamstring Stretch: Sit on the floor, one leg extended and the other bent. Reach toward the toes of the extended leg while keeping your back straight. Hold for 30 seconds then switch sides

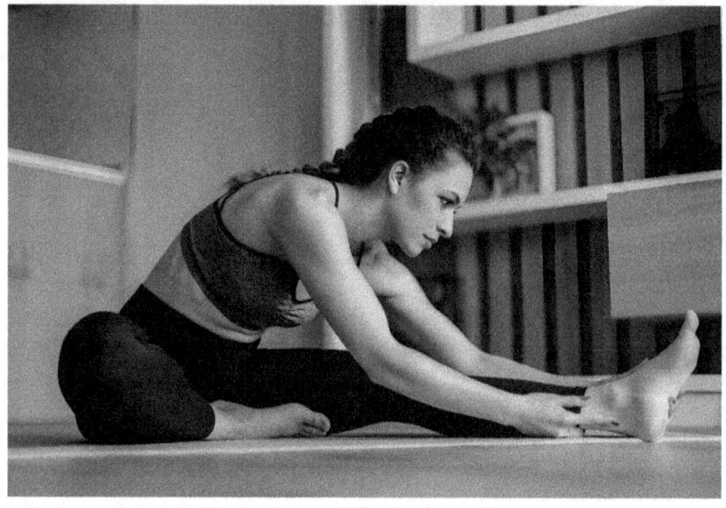

4. Quad Stretch: Stand and balance by grasping a wall or a chair. Bend one knee and hold your ankle in your hand. Pull your heel toward your glutes until you feel a stretch

at the front of your thigh. Hold for 30 seconds then switch sides.

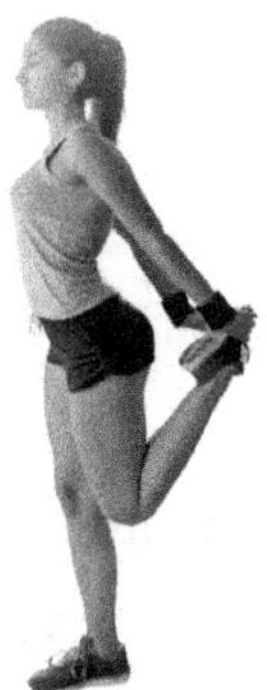

5. Inner Thigh Stretch: Sit on the floor, legs extended. Open your legs as wide as you can, then bend forward from the hips until you feel a stretch in your inner thighs. Hold for 30 seconds.

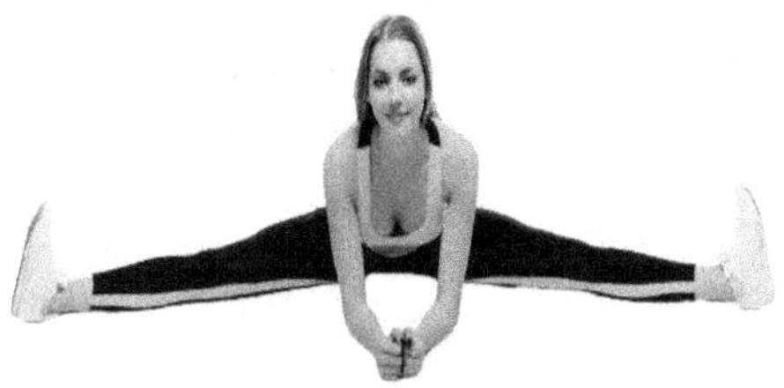

Tips For Effective Stretching:

- Always warm up your muscles before stretching to avoid injury.

- Hold Each Stretch: Give each stretch 20-30 seconds to enable the muscles to relax and lengthen.

- Remember to breathe deeply and gently while stretching to help relax your muscles.

- Don't Overdo It: Stretch until you feel slight discomfort, not pain. Overstretching might cause harm.

Regular stretching exercises can greatly benefit your glutes, hips, and thighs by increasing flexibility, mobility, and general muscular health. Stretching for just a few minutes every day can improve your performance, minimize your risk of injury, and make you feel more comfortable and safe in your actions.

Cooldown: The Importance of Cooling Down After Workout

Picture this! You just finished a grueling workout. Your heart is racing, your muscles are tired, and you're covered in sweat. It's tempting to collapse on the floor and call it a day, but there's one crucial phase you shouldn't overlook: the cooldown.

The cooldown is analogous to the gradual descent after reaching the summit of a mountain. It is your body's natural mechanism for gradually returning to a state of rest and recovery after exertion. Just as you wouldn't jump from the top to the valley below, you shouldn't go straight from intense exercise to utter relaxation without a cooldown.

So, why is cooldown so important?

1. Aids in Recovery: After a workout, your muscles are weary and likely damaged from the stress of exercise. A cooldown allows your muscles to relax and recover, reducing the likelihood of pain and injury.

2. Prevents Blood Pooling: During activity, blood is rapidly pumped to the working muscles. A sudden stop may cause blood to pool in the extremities, resulting in lightheadedness or fainting. A cooldown helps to gradually restore blood flow to normal levels.

3. Reduces Muscle Stiffness: Cooling down helps keep the muscles from becoming stiff and tight after heavy exercise. It increases flexibility and range of motion, making it easier to move and operate after a workout.

4. Aids in Waste Removal: Exercise generates waste products in the muscles, such as lactic acid. A cooldown helps to flush out these waste products by keeping the blood flowing and increasing circulation.

5. Promotes Mental Relaxation: A cooldown may be a calming and meditative experience, allowing you to mentally decompress after a strenuous workout. It can also help to lower your heart rate and provide a sense of well-being.

6. Improves training consistency: Making the cooldown a regular part of your routine increases your chances of sticking to your training plan. It sends a signal to your body that the work

out is over, allowing you to psychologically return to normal life.

Including a cooldown does not have to make your training regimen more difficult. After your main workout, do 5-10 minutes of gentle walking or running, followed by some mild stretching. The solution is to listen to your body's cues and give it the time and care it needs to heal itself.

Don't skip the cooldown the next time you work out. Consider it a critical component of your training strategy, similar to the warm-up. You'll be one step closer to meeting your fitness goals, and your body will thank you.

Nutritious Tips for Muscle Building and Toning

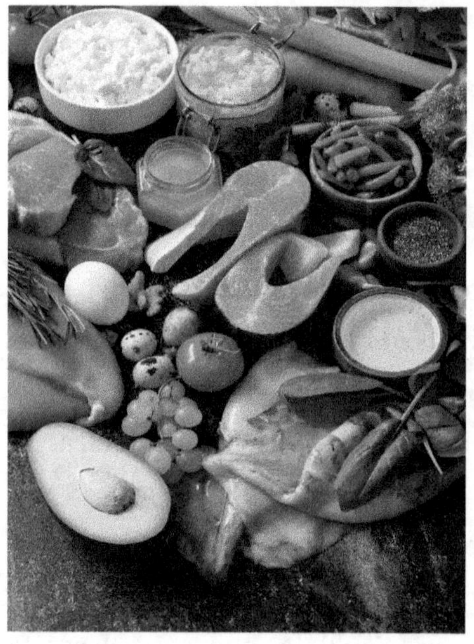

Muscle growth and toning require more than just weight lifting and aerobics. Nutrition is essential for providing the energy and nutrients needed for muscle growth and repair. You can adjust your diet to support your fitness goals and get a toned and sculpted figure by following these basic nutritional recommendations.

1. Protein-rich foods: Because protein is the foundation of muscle tissue, it is critical to ingest adequate amounts regularly. Lean protein options for your meals include tofu, dairy products, fish, chicken, and lentils.

2. Balanced meal: Make sure your food has an appropriate fat and carbohydrate ratio in addition to protein. While healthy fats help to produce hormones and improve overall health, carbohydrates give energy for exercise.

3. Meal Timing: Consume a well-balanced lunch with carbohydrates and protein within one to two hours of exercising. This provides you with the energy you need to exercise, as well as the nutrients your muscles require to grow and repair.

4. Hydrated: Staying properly hydrated is essential for strong muscles and overall health. Throughout the day, drink plenty of water, especially before, during, and after heavy activity.

5. Nutrient-Dense Foods: Pay special attention to eating whole, high-nutrient foods including fruits, vegetables, whole grains, and lean meats. Essential vitamins, minerals, and antioxidants included in these foods improve overall health and muscle function.

6. Supplements: To improve muscle growth and recovery, consider including protein powder, creatine, and branched-chain amino acids (BCAAs) in your diet. However, before starting a new supplement regimen, always seek medical advice.

7. Portion Control: Be mindful of serving sizes to avoid overindulging in food and consuming unnecessary calories. Use a food scale or measuring glasses to ensure you're eating enough to meet your goals.

8. Consistency: When it comes to fitness and nutrition, consistency is essential. To achieve the best long-term results, stick to your diet and exercise routine.

You may efficiently strengthen and tone your muscles, giving your body a stronger, more toned appearance, by following these nutritional suggestions in conjunction with a steady workout schedule. Remember that maintaining your overall level of fitness is dependent on more than just what you accomplish at the gym. It also depends on what you put into your body.

Protein-Rich Foods for Muscle Growth and Recovery

Protein is required for muscle growth and recovery during physical exertion. During exercise, your muscles incur microscopic tears, which protein helps to rebuild and heal while also strengthening and reinforcing.

The Role of Protein in Muscle Growth and Recovery

1. Muscle Repair: Protein provides amino acids, or building blocks, that are required to heal damaged muscle tissue. Your muscles require these amino acids to repair and strengthen after an activity.

2. muscular expansion: The process of muscular hypertrophy, or muscle enlargement, is protein-dependent. Gaining muscle mass necessitates increasing muscle protein synthesis, which is aided by consuming adequate protein.

3. Less Muscle Soreness: Eating adequate protein will help reduce muscle soreness after an exercise, allowing for faster recovery and better preparation for the next one.

Protein-Rich Foods for Muscle Growth

1. Chicken breast:

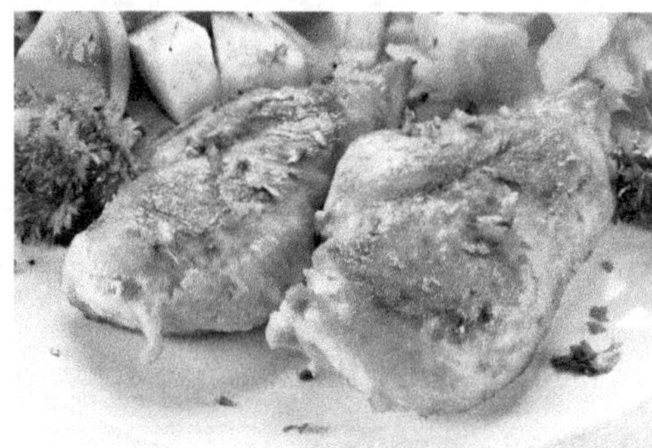

Chicken breast is an excellent choice for muscle building and recovery because it is a lean protein source with a high protein quality and low-fat content.

2. Fish: Omega-3 fatty acids, which are high in protein and have anti-inflammatory properties that can aid in muscle regeneration, are found in mackerel, salmon, and tuna.

3. Eggs: With all nine essential amino acids, eggs provide a complete protein source. They are also a great source of nutrients including choline, which is essential for strong muscles.

4. Greek Yogurt: High in protein and probiotics, Greek yogurt helps aid digestion and nutrition absorption, promoting muscle regeneration.

5. Quinoa:

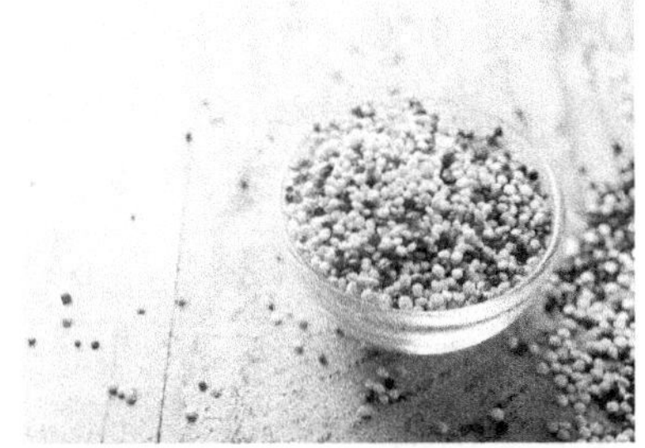

Quinoa is a complete protein that provides energy through complex carbs. This is an excellent choice for vegans and vegetarians looking to increase their protein intake.

6. Beans and Legumes: Beans and legumes, such as chickpeas, lentils, and black beans, are high in protein and fiber, making them an excellent choice for muscular strength and recovery.

7. Lean Beef:

Iron and protein are
essential for the body
to carry oxygen to the
muscles and
produce lean beef cuts
such as tenderloin and
sirloin.

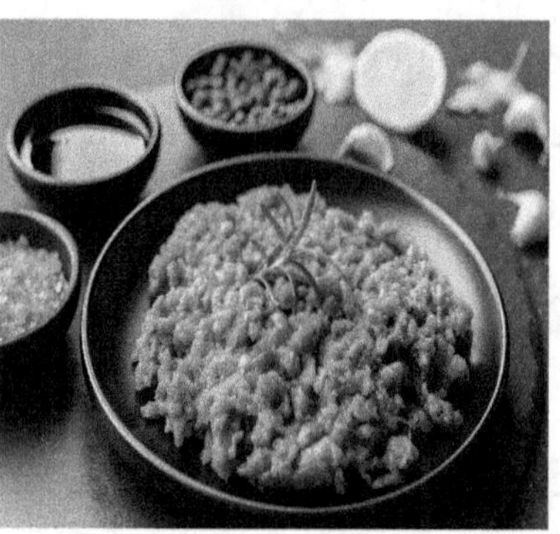

Including Protein in Your Food:

Aim to consume a source of protein in every meal and snack to maximize muscle building and recovery. This can assist in making sure you consume enough protein throughout the day to help you reach your muscle-building objectives. To ensure your muscles have the nutrition they require for growth and repair, try eating a protein-rich snack or meal no later than one hour after your workout.

Since it provides the building blocks needed for muscle repair and rebuilding after exercise, protein is crucial for both muscular growth and recovery. Consuming a diet high in protein can support your overall health and fitness objectives as well as help you get the most out of your muscle-building efforts.

Water Hydration: Your Workout's Unsung Hero

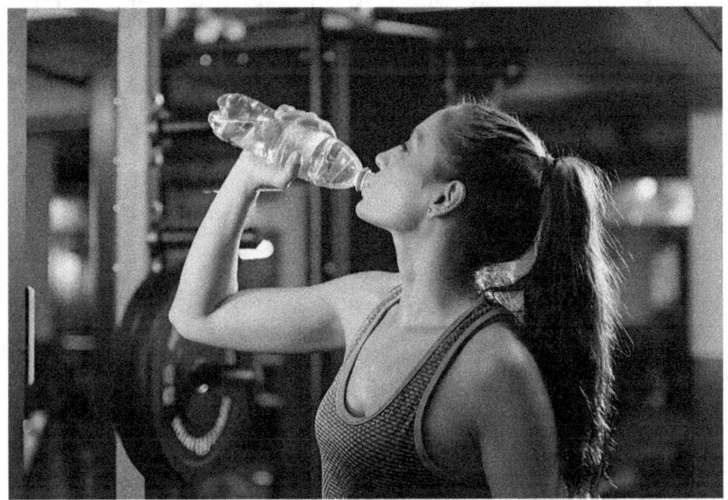

Consider this: Halfway into your workout, you're pushing through the perspiration and feeling the burn. Your body is screaming for water above all else while your heart is racing, your muscles are straining, and your body is working hard.

In the world of fitness, water is frequently disregarded, yet it is the unsung hero that maintains your body functioning at its peak, particularly while you work. It's critical for your performance, recuperation, and general health to stay hydrated when exercising.

Why Is Hydration Vital When Working Out?

1. Preserve Fluid Balance: Your body loses electrolytes and fluids as you perspire. By keeping these vital chemicals in balance while exercising, you can avoid dehydration and the negative impact it can have on your performance.

2. Controls Body Temperature: Your body naturally cools itself through sweat. Maintaining enough hydration helps control body temperature, which helps you avoid overheating when doing out hard.

3. Supports Muscle Function: Weariness and cramping in the muscles can result from dehydration. Your muscles will get the oxygen and nutrients they require to perform at their best if you stay properly hydrated.

4. Performance Enhancement: Drinking enough water before, during, and after exercise will help you perform

better overall and with strength and endurance. Your training intensity and duration might be adversely affected by even minor dehydration.

5. Encourages Recovery: Refueling with water after exercise aids in the process of healing. It can lessen stiffness and discomfort in your muscles, enabling you to recover more quickly for your next workout.

How to Drink Enough Water When Exercising:

1. Sip Plenty of Water: Make sure to stay hydrated before, during, and after your exercise. To stay hydrated without packing on the pounds, drink water regularly.

2. Take Into Account Electrolyte Drinks: If you're exercising hard or for extended periods, you should think about sports drinks that replace the electrolytes you lose through perspiration.

3. Pay Attention to the Color of Your pee: Light yellow pee suggests enough hydration, whereas darker urine may indicate dehydration.

4. Pay Attention to Your Body: Your body needs extra water when you're thirsty. When you are thirsty, don't ignore it; sip water.

5. Make a Plan: Make sure you're well-hydrated before working out, particularly if you'll be working out in the heat or for a longer amount of time.

Staying hydrated is crucial for your performance, recuperation, and general well-being during your workout. Giving your body the water it requires will guarantee that every drop of perspiration brings you one step closer to your fitness objectives. Thus, remember to drink as though your workout depended on it the next time you hit the gym or put on your running shoes—because it does.

Motivation for Persistent Fitness Pursuit

It's admirable to start a fitness adventure because it can make you happy and healthier. It can be difficult at times to remain dedicated and motivated on this path, though. It's crucial to acknowledge the progress you've made along the way and to remind yourself of the reasons you started for these reasons.

Setting Achievable Goals: Having attainable goals is essential to maintaining motivation while pursuing a fitness regimen. These objectives must be time-bound, meaningful, quantifiable, attainable, and specific (SMART). Rather than declaring, "I want to lose weight," for instance, you may make your aim to "lose 1-2 pounds per week by exercising for 30 minutes a day and eating a balanced diet."

Monitoring Your Progress: Monitoring your advancement is an additional useful strategy for maintaining motivation. Keeping track of your progress, whether through a journal, fitness app, or even just writing it on a calendar, may be quite motivating. Appreciate your incremental gains—such as going the additional mile or lifting bigger weights—because they all add up to your total development.

Identifying Your Motivation: There are varying reasons why people decide to embark on a fitness journey. When motivation starts to wane, it's critical to remind yourself of these goals, whether they be to enhance your appearance, increase your confidence, or simply feel better about your health. To keep yourself motivated, surround yourself with great role models in the fitness industry as well as encouraging friends and family.

Building a Support Network: Having a network of people to lean on will help you stay motivated tremendously. Having others who support and understand your journey can help you stay accountable and motivated, whether you're working out with a workout partner, enrolling in a fitness class, or engaging in online groups.

Embracing the path: Lastly, it's critical to keep in mind that the path to fitness is about more than simply getting to a goal; it's also about appreciating the journey itself. Celebrate your victories, accept the ups and downs, and take lessons from your failures. You are moving in the right way with each step you take to lead a healthier lifestyle.

It takes commitment, perseverance, and a positive outlook to stay inspired on your fitness path. You may stay motivated and keep moving forward toward a healthier you by setting reasonable goals, monitoring your development, discovering your motivation, assembly
in a support network, and appreciating the trip.

Conclusion

In conclusion, focusing your exercise regimen on your glutes, hips, and thighs can help you develop a stronger, more balanced lower body, which will enhance your general health and fitness. You may increase functional movement, lower your chance of injury, and improve your athletic performance by including exercises that focus on specific muscle groups. A well-planned warm-up is also necessary to prime your body for activity, lower your chance of injury, and improve your performance. You may maximize your workout and reach your fitness objectives by setting aside time to properly warm up and concentrate on these important muscle groups.